The Book
on
Osteoarthritis Treatment

By
Nathan Wei, MD, FACP, FACR

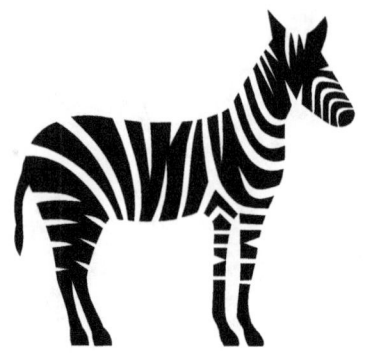

Library of Congress Cataloging-in-Publication Data pending
Wei, Nathan

Key words: 1. Arthritis Treatment 2. Osteoarthritis

This book should not be a substitute for a thorough examination by your physician. The products that are mentioned in this book are recommended. Prior to using any of them, we recommend you seek advice from a qualified specialist. Neither the publisher nor the author may be held liable for any injury, loss, or damage sustained by anyone who relies on the information contained in the book.

Table of Contents

Chapter 1 5

Introduction 5

Chapter 2 7

How Does Osteoarthritis Develop? 7

Chapter 3 12

Symptoms of Osteoarthritis 12

Chapter 4 19

Diagnosis 19

Chapter 5 21

Treatment 21

Chapter 6 90

Conclusion 90

Chapter 1

Introduction

"My daughter's birthday wish was to go to an amusement park, but my knees hurt too much to take her." Those are the words of a patient of mine a couple of years ago. Over the last 25 years, though, I've heard countless variations of this lament. Sometimes, it's the knees; other times, it's the hips or low back. But whatever the complaint, these people are describing an affliction called osteoarthritis (OA).

"Yeah, Uncle Joe had 'Arthur' pretty bad. His knees were bowed..."

Osteoarthritis is the most common form of arthritis. It's the one that we all picture when somebody says, "I have arthritis."

Approximately 50 million Americans suffer from arthritis. That figure comes from the Communicable Disease Center in Atlanta, but it's probably an underestimation. It is estimated that 70 million Americans will suffer from arthritis by the year 2020. A significant percentage of those patients will suffer from osteoarthritis.

Arthritic symptoms account for the majority of physician visits in patients over the age of 65. It remains the most common cause of disability. And again the most likely type of arthritis leading to these issues is osteoarthritis.

Chapter 2

How Does Osteoarthritis Develop?

A normal joint consists of two bones that interact with each other. The ends of the bones are covered by a thin layer of cartilage, and the joint is enclosed in a joint capsule that is lined by a layer of cells called synoviocytes. Referred to collectively as the synovium, these synoviocytes produce a small amount of lubricant called synovial fluid that allows the joint surfaces to glide easily.

The structure of cartilage provides a clue as to how osteoarthritis develops. Cartilage, the gristle at the end of long bones, functions as a cushion—a shock absorber. It also allows the smooth gliding motion of joints. During joint loading, cartilage compresses. Then…when the load is removed, it reverts to its normal thickness.

Cartilage is made of two components: cells and a matrix. The cells, called chondrocytes, sit inside the extracellular matrix—much like grapes sitting inside gelatin. The matrix, which is made by the chondrocytes, consists of fluid (mostly water) and a framework made up of collagen, proteoglycans, and glycoproteins.

The purpose of the matrix is to give cartilage elastic properties.

Up until recently, it was assumed that osteoarthritis was primarily the result of a simple wear-and-tear process. However, there is growing evidence that osteoarthritis is actually a repair response to the normal wear and tear that occurs in all joints.

Under normal circumstances, when cartilage is injured there is a repair process that compensates for the injury. So... there is a regulated balance between cartilage degradation and cartilage repair.

Unfortunately, at some point in time repair cannot keep up with damage. This may be because of genetic factors... or it may be due to the magnitude of injury to joint cartilage. Nonetheless, the end result is that cartilage wears away more than it can be repaired.

Some researchers have termed this phenomenon, "joint failure".

Cartilage itself does not have blood vessels nor does it have nerve fibers. So the pain that accompanies osteoarthritis is due to a complex interplay between local inflammation which contributes to the damage from OA (Pettipher ER, Higgs GA, Henderson B. Interleukin-1 induces leukocyte infiltration and cartilage proteoglycan degradation in the synovial joint. Proc Natl Acad Sci USA. 1986; 83: 8749-8753.) as well as mechanical factors.

These mechanical factors include such things as irritation of the joint capsule as a result of bone spurs, as well as loss of mechanical integrity of the joint because of ligament stretching, muscle spasm, and so on.

While the most commonly affected joints are weight-bearing areas such as the neck, low back, hips, and knees, other areas where there is a significant amount of joint stress such as the base of the thumb and big toe are also affected.

Finally, there is also a type of osteoarthritis that selectively attacks the fingers. This appears to be more common in women than men.

Risk factors for OA include a family history of the disease, older age, trauma to the joint, excessive weight, repetitive motion, and the presence of other types of arthritis.

Many people who have osteoarthritis don't know that they have it. Some of these people have minor aches and pains that they ignore. Others are symptom-free! Osteoarthritis symptoms typically begin after the age of 40, although the development of the disease obviously begins much earlier—possibly as early as the teens.

This is how osteoarthritis develops...

In the first phase of OA, the matrix begins to accumulate water as a result of damage to the collagen network. This leads to swelling of the cartilage. There is also an increase in the synthesis of proteoglycans, the substance that give cartilage its elasticity. This is an attempt by the chondrocytes to repair damage. The chondrocytes can't keep up the pace. The result is a change in the composition of the matrix framework. There is a loss of chondrocytes at the surface of the

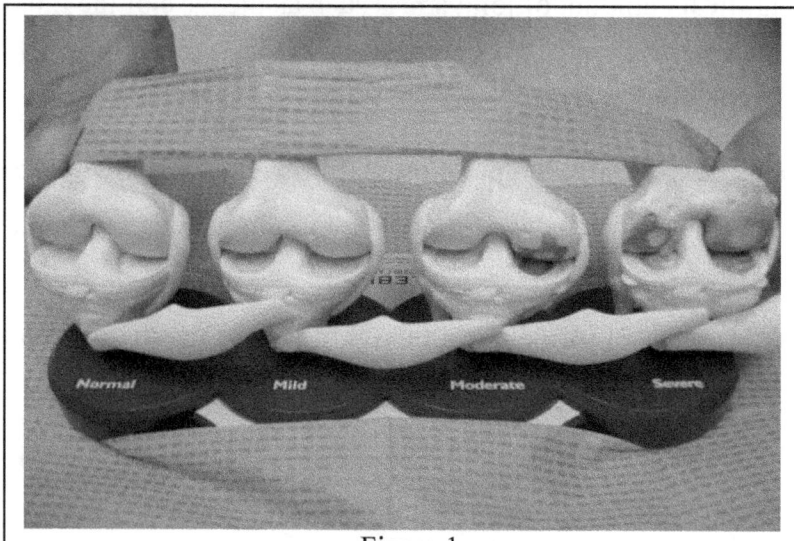

Figure 1
Progression of osteoarthritis from normal on the
left to severe on the right

cartilage, while the deeper layers try to produce more chondrocytes to replace those that have been lost. Unfortunately, this is a losing battle, and both the substance of the matrix and the number of chondrocytes decline. This leads to softening and flaking (called fibrillation) of the cartilage. The chondrocytes then begin to produce enzymes that cause further cartilage damage. (Figure 1)

At the same time, the underlying bone begins to harden, thicken, and form holes (called cysts) under the cartilage. The bone also starts to form bony spurs (called osteophytes). Bits of cartilage and bone flake off.

The lining of the joint (synovium) becomes inflamed. The inflammation produces chemical messengers called cytokines that further damage cartilage, bone, and other structures within the joint. The major cytokines that seem to play a role in OA are tumor necrosis factor-alpha and interleukin 1 (IL-1). In addition to these cytokines, there are other substances that have roles in the inflammation associated with OA, including matrix metalloprotease, prostaglandins, and nitric oxide. The result is that chondrocytes undergo premature, programmed death (this is called apoptosis), and cartilage degradation progresses.

Chapter 3

Symptoms of Osteoarthritis

The most common symptom of OA is pain. Multiple factors contribute to the pain: increased pressure and possibly microfractures inside the bone underneath the diseased cartilage, irritation of the tissue surrounding the bone (called the periosteum), bony spurs, shrinking of the joint capsule, inflammation of the joint capsule and synovium, irritation of the ligaments around the joint, spasm of muscle, and muscle fatigue. Night pain often occurs in those patients who have an inflammatory component to their OA.

Stiffness is also common among patients with OA, although the severity of stiffness is less than that among patients with rheumatoid arthritis. Stiffness in the morning generally lasts less than 1 hour. Because inactivity generally makes stiffness worse, patients may get stiff if they sit for a long period of time (e.g., on an automobile trip).

Night pain is common in those patients who have an inflammatory component to their osteoarthritis.

How pain is felt in different areas...

Osteoarthritis pain can range from being a nuisance to being intolerable.

The pain from osteoarthritis can cause a wide variety of pain syndromes depending on the location.

Since one of its primary functions is to support the entire skeleton, the spinal column is often affected by osteoarthritis.

The spinal column consists of bones (vertebrae) that are stacked, one upon the other, and separated from each other by discs in the front and facet joints in the back. The spinal cord runs from the brain down the spinal column to the low back in a tunnel called the spinal canal. Between each vertebra, the spinal cord sends out a pair of nerve roots, one to the left, the other to the right.

When osteoarthritis develops in the spinal column, it is characterized by gradual loss of water content in the discs which causes them to dry out and flatten out.

At the same time arthritis develops in the facet joints. The end result is narrowing of the spinal canal as well as narrowing of the openings for the nerve roots where they exit from the spinal cord.

Osteoarthritis in the neck is often described early by patients as a grating, grinding sensation in their neck when they turn their heads. Almost like there's "sand in there."

When pain occurs it can be localized to the neck.

When nerve roots that exit the spinal cord are irritated, the result is localized pain and muscle spasm. That's why many patients with neck arthritis will have pain that travels up the back of the head or radiates into the area between the shoulder blades. Sometimes the pain will radiate down the arm. In fact, osteoarthritis of the neck can be responsible for pain that is felt anywhere from the crown of the head to mid chest - front or back!

Osteoarthritis in the mid-spine will usually cause pain in the mid-spine or it can radiate to one side or the other, particularly if there is a lot of muscle spasm.

Osteoarthritis in the low back will cause either localized low back pain or it can cause sciatica… pain that radiates down the leg. The pain may be accompanied by numbness and tingling. In advanced cases when the arthritis causes significant narrowing of the spinal canal, the spinal cord becomes compressed to the point that the patient will walk in a bent over posture since straightening up causes the pain in the back to worsen. The patient may also complain of an aching and cramping sensation in their legs when they walk. The aching and cramping is alleviated by sitting down for a few minutes, only to return when the patient walks again. This is the typical pain pattern of a patient who has spinal stenosis - narrowing of the spinal canal due to osteoarthritis. In extreme cases, there is loss of bladder and bowel function. This is considered a neurosurgical emergency.

Patients with osteoarthritis of the hip tend to have groin pain. Sometimes, they also have buttock pain. Pain from osteoarthritis of the hip may be referred down the front of the thigh to the knee. Also, patients with osteoarthritis of the hip may have trouble going up and down stairs, getting into and out of chairs, and even tying and untying their shoes as well as putting on their shoes and socks. These patients may hold their hip slightly flexed. Pain at night is often present.

Patients with osteoarthritis of the knees may be either bow-legged or knock-kneed (Figure 2). Locking, clicking, and even a sensation of "give-way" may be noted. Patients will often have an effusion (fluid) in the knee joint. Night pain is frequent. Stiffness in the knees occurs with inactivity (eg, sitting down for a long time, then getting up to walk).

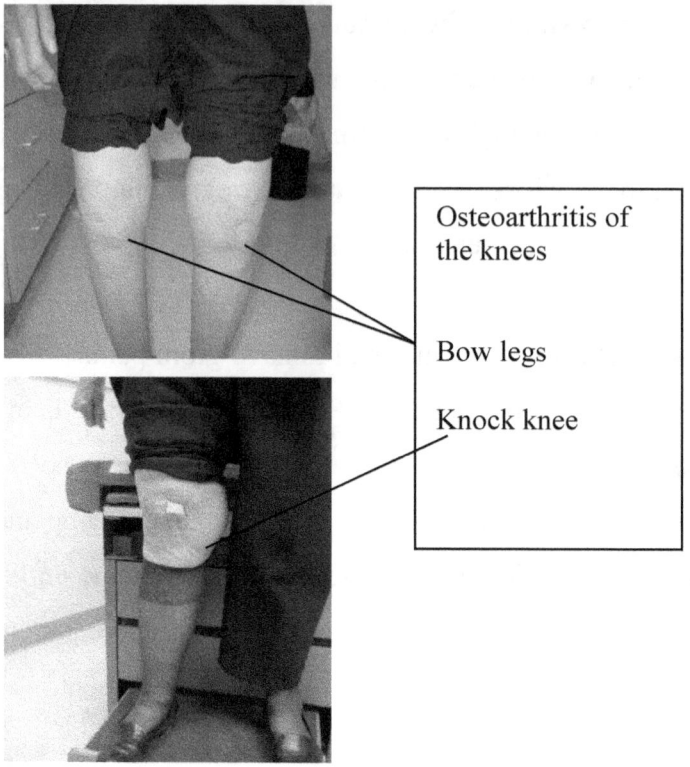

Osteoarthritis of
the knees

Bow legs

Knock knee

Figure 2

Signs of OA include joint swelling and tenderness with pressure applied to the affected joint. The range of motion is often restricted. Joint deformity indicates advanced disease; loss of function indicates even more advanced disease.

In addition to stiffness, patients who have osteoarthritis in the hands may have difficulty making a fist.

Osteoarthritis in the hands presents with swelling and pain involving the row of joints furthest from the palms. These joints are called the distal interphalangeal joints (DIPs). And the bumps that form here are called Heberden's nodes (Figure 3). The next row closer to the palms are the proximal interphalangeal joints (PIPs). The bumps that form here are called Bouchard's nodes (see Figure 3). Some patients have pain and possibly grinding at the base of the thumb.

Some patients, particularly women will have an aggressive form of osteoarthritis which is called "inflammatory erosive osteoarthritis" (Figure 3).

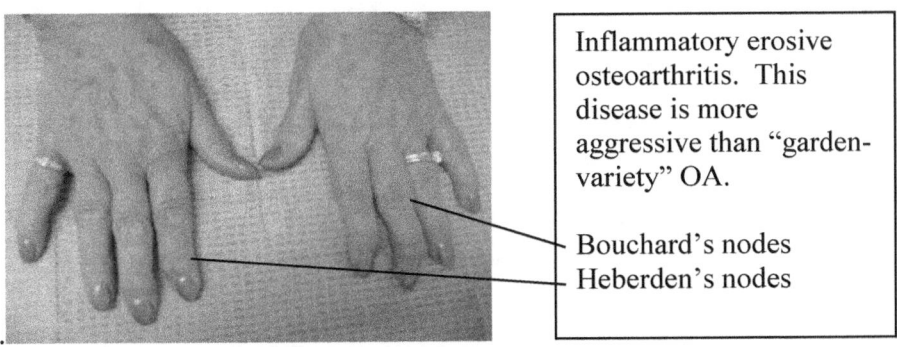

Inflammatory erosive osteoarthritis. This disease is more aggressive than "garden-variety" OA.

Bouchard's nodes
Heberden's nodes

Figure 3

The other common area for osteoarthritis to develop is the big toe joint. When wearing away of the cartilage is pronounced and also accompanied by inflammation of the bursa (fluid-filled cushion) next to the toe, a patient will develop what is called, a bunion.

While the most commonly affected areas have been described above, osteoarthritis can affect virtually any joint in the body. For example, osteoarthritis of the jaw joint can cause "TMJ syndrome."

Osteoarthritis of the shoulder can develop as a result of trauma. The same can be said for osteoarthritis of the ankle. And so on.

The severity of symptoms and signs doesn't necessarily correlate with the stage of disease (as measured by the amount of cartilage loss)! Some patients with severe disease have few symptoms, while other patients who have only moderate disease can suffer from a great deal of pain, as well as a very limited range of motion of the joint.

Chapter 4

Diagnosis

The history suggests the diagnosis, and the physical examination confirms it. In addition to pain, careful attention is paid to physical function, global status (e.g., How are you doing?), quality of life, and the ability to perform different tasks.

Although laboratory tests aren't particularly helpful in making the diagnosis of osteoarthritis, they do help in excluding other types of arthritis. X-ray films help confirm the diagnosis of OA. Unfortunately, however, x-ray films are not useful in finding early OA; changes on an x-ray film are a late finding. Standing knee x-ray films are particularly useful in indicating whether a patient should consider surgery sooner rather than later.

Magnetic resonance imaging (MRI) may be more helpful than x-ray films in the diagnosis of OA. However, even MRI is not that effective in detecting early OA. Arthroscopy (looking inside the joint with a small telescope inserted into the knee) seems to be the most sensitive technique. We recently completed an arthroscopy study involving volunteers who had no symptoms of OA, normal x-ray films, and normal MRI studies. Of the eight "healthy" volunteers, four had grade

2 OA (on a scale of 4 with 4 being the most severe) and two had stage 3! (Unpublished data)

Chapter 5

Treatment

The goals of therapy are to reduce pain, improve function, slow down the progression of disease (if possible), control co-morbidities (other medical conditions that may play a role in the outcome of the disease) and improve quality of life.

Non - traditional treatment
Supplements:

What if you could take a natural vitamin preparation that would help you with osteoarthritis? Well, perhaps you can...

Science is finding therapeutic potential in dietary supplements. The problem is... where do you find the right information and type of supplement that is best for you?

What it boils down to is finding the supplement that is best suited to your needs. If you have arthritis or any other chronic condition and want a natural approach, or want to avoid side-effects from prescription medicines, or just want to hedge your bets...this chapter is for you.

Supplements come from three major sources: plants, animals, or they can be synthesized in the lab.

Most supplements don't have the luxury of having had strictly controlled scientific studies to bolster their claims.

Pharmaceuticals do...because pharmaceutical manufacturers must test their products over and over again to prove safety and efficacy to the Food and Drug Administration.

Supplements don't because they're not regulated by the FDA - and because it's difficult to perform a supplement study requiring large numbers of patients. It's also important to remember that because supplements come in different forms - what is available to you may not be the same supplement studied in the clinical trials.

So long-term safety is always an issue, just like it is with regular drugs!

And supplements often have side-effects that are not well known.

Nonetheless, here is a rundown of the herbs and supplements that might interest you.

ASU. This is a compound consisting of extracts derived from one-third avocado oil and two-thirds soybean oil after hydrolysis. There is evidence that these ingredients might stimulate collagen synthesis in culture.

Four double blind clinical trials with a total of 751 randomized patients compared ASU (usually 300 mg once a day) with placebo in people with osteoarthritis of knee or hip. All used recommended procedures for osteoarthritis trials, and all patients randomized into the studies had osteoarthritis, pain of at least moderate intensity, and were using NSAIDS (non-steroidal anti-inflammatory drugs) for pain control or had established pain of at least six months duration.

All four trials had similar outcomes, measuring pain, function, NSAID use and patient global outcome, and incorporated adverse events and withdrawals. One study had a primary outcome of x-ray joint space narrowing. Duration was three months in two, six to eight months in one, and 24 months in the fourth. Three trials had better pain and function with ASU + NSAID compared with placebo + NSAID over three to six months. In all three, better pain relief was achieved with a lower dose of NSAID. Both these effects took several months to develop. A fourth trial showed no difference in pain, function, or daily NSAID use over 24 months.

Bioflavonoids: The plant-derived bioflavonoids, often found in combination with vitamin C, have strong antioxidant and anti-inflammatory properties and appear to moderate key enzyme reactions in inflammation. Bioflavonoids also affect the structure of collagen—

the strong fibrous protein found in all connective tissue including cartilage. Bioflavonoids affect collagen structure by protecting it from free radical destruction and by cross-linking directly with the collagen fibers. Bioflavonoids can also prove helpful in correcting capillary fragility in the brain, which can lead to what are known as "mini-strokes." Other problems related to capillary fragility, like bruising very easily, can generally improved with the dietary supplementation of bioflavonoids. An anti-inflammatory compound that has been shown in a number of double-blind placebo controlled studies to be effective for osteoarthritis is currently available. It is called Limbrel.

Black currant oil (*Ribes officinalis*): Major source of ALA (alpha-linoleic acid) and GLA (gamma-linolenic acid). ALA is an omega-3 fatty acid that, to a limited extent, can be converted in the body into two other important omega-3s — EPA (eicosapentaenoic acid) and DHA (docosahexaenoic acid). GLA is an omega-6 fatty acid. The body ordinarily is able to produce sufficient GLA from the essential fatty acid linoleic acid (LA), which is found in foods containing oils from corn, sunflower, safflower, soy, peanut and other plants, including flaxseed.

However, GLA production may be reduced in several conditions (advanced age, diabetes, high alcohol intake, eczema, cyclic mastitis, viral infections, excessive saturated fat intake, elevated cholesterol, and some vitamin/mineral deficiencies). In such cases, supplements may be beneficial. Seed oils from black currant, borage, and evening primrose are among the few that are rich in GLA.

Mediterranean diets, which are associated with a lower risk of coronary artery disease and certain types of cancer, are high in ALA. However, the beneficial effects of EPA and DHA (which include cardiovascular benefits and reduced pain associated with rheumatoid arthritis and menstrual cramps) have not been seen with ALA alone. Black currant oil, which has mixture of both ALA and GLA may, consequently, have anti-inflammatory effects due to its GLA content.

GLA may be useful in diseases that involve inflammation. It may also have some benefit in treating rheumatoid arthritis (especially as purified GLA and when combined with traditional treatments) and Raynaud's phenomenon. Many other potential uses, including some in conjunction with fish oils, have been explored, but evidence is either weak or very preliminary. Although studies in osteoarthritis are lacking, I don't see why this preparation would not be effective for the condition.

Black currant seed oil has the ability to reduce prostaglandin production. (Wu D, et al. Am J Clin Nutr 1999 Oct; 70(4):536-43). This contains 6-19 percent gamma-linolenic acid (GLA). GLA is an omega-6 fatty acid that has potent anti-inflammatory properties. This lessens joint pain and stiffness as well as swelling. One placebo-controlled trial in 56 patients with rheumatoid arthritis showed that patients taking GLA for 6 months had significant improvement in joint pain, stiffness, and grip strength (Belch JJ, et al. *Ann Rheum Dis* 1988;47:96-104). GLA was safe. GLA can thin the blood so if you're on a blood thinner, use caution. Again, the lack of studies in osteoarthritis make me somewhat hesitant to recommend this but the anti-inflammatory effect is compelling.

Borage oil comes from the borage plant. Borage is an annual plant that grows wild in the Mediterranean countries and is cultivated elsewhere. The hollow, bristly, branched and spreading stem grows up to two feet tall. It contains 20-26 percent of the fatty acid GLA. Oils containing the omega-6 fatty acid gamma linolenic acid (GLA)— borage oil (Pullman-Mooar S, et al. *Arthritis Rheum* 1990; 33:1526–1533; Leventhal LJ, et al. *Ann Intern Med* 993;119:867–73; Zurier RB, et al. *Arthritis Rheum* 1996; 39:1808-17)—have been reported to be effective in the treatment for people with RA. The effects are similar to that for black currant oil, i.e., it has anti-inflammatory properties). (See GLA.)

Boswellia has anti-inflammatory properties that have been compared to those of the NSAIDS used by many for inflammatory conditions. Clinical trials in humans using boswellia alone are lacking. However, one clinical trial found that a combination of boswellia, ashwagandha, turmeric, and zinc effectively treated pain and stiffness associated with osteoarthritis but did not improve joint health, according to X-rays of the affected joint. Unlike NSAIDs, however, long-term use of boswellia does not lead to irritation or ulceration of the stomach (Safayhi H. *J Pharmacol Exp Ther* 1992; 261:1143-6; Kulkarni RR, *J Ethnopharmacol* 1991; 33:91-5).

Bromelain is an enzyme derived from pineapples and is important for pain - free movement of joints. Bromelain is an anti-inflammatory that has been shown to reduce joint swelling but without any side effects. How does it help? Bromelain *(Anas comosus)* inhibits "bad" prostaglandin production and reduces inflammation (*Japanese Journal of Pharmacology*, 1972, vol. 22). Bromelain has long been a mainstay for treating muscle injuries (Blonstein J. *Practitioner* 1960; 203:206), yet now it is believed its anti-inflammatory actions may also ease arthritic pain. The enzymes obtained from the stem of the pineapple plant *(Ananas comosus)* help break down scar tissue, decrease tissue fluid called edema, and block inflammation (Ako H, et al. *Arch Int Pharmacodynamics* 1981; 254:157-67).

Boron: This is an essential trace mineral needed for healthy muscle and joint tissue. Boron is renowned for its role in helping to prevent or slow the effects of osteoporosis. (Newnham RE. *Int Clin Nutr Rev* 1991; 11:68-70 [letter]).

Boron, though not an antioxidant, does help prevent cells from releasing free radicals. Epidemiologic studies show that people in countries with low amounts of boron in the soil often have osteoarthritis. (De Fabio A. *Townsend Letter for Doctors* 1990 Feb-

Mar: 143-8.) Boron supplementation may also encourage cartilage repair and synthesis. One open trial demonstrated that daily boron supplementation caused symptom remission in 90 percent of arthritis patients studied, including people with osteoarthritis, rheumatoid arthritis and juvenile arthritis (Newnham RE. *Int Clin Nutr Rev* 1991;11: 68-70).

Cat's claw (*Uncaria tomentosa*) Bark from a woody vine that grows in the Amazon rain forest. Oxyindole alkaloids appear to give this plant much of its activity, particularly as a stimulant for the immune system. The alkaloids and other constituents, such as glycosides, may account for the anti-inflammatory and anti-oxidant actions of this herb. It has been used traditionally for osteoarthritis.

In a double-blind trial, 100 mg per day of a freeze-dried preparation of cat's claw taken for four weeks was significantly more effective than a placebo at relieving pain and improving the overall condition (Piscoya J, et al. *Inflamm Res* 2001;50:442-8.) One study showed this compound to reduce knee pain in OA (Sandoval-Chacon M, et al. *Ailment Pharmacol Ther* 1998; 12:1279-1289). It can cause headaches, nausea, and dizziness, along with a drop in blood pressure. There is some evidence to suggest it may aggravate autoimmune diseases.

Cayenne pepper: This contains capsaicin which helps release endorphins, the body's natural pain relievers. It also blocks substance

P, a chemical responsible for pain transmission (Rains C. *Drugs Aging*. 1995; 7:317-28). It's most often used as a topical agent and is effective for osteoarthritis of the knee. A cream containing small amounts of capsaicin, a substance found in cayenne pepper, can help relieve pain when rubbed onto arthritic joints, according to the results of a double-blind trial. (Deal CL. *Clin Ther* 1991; 13:383–95). Capsaicin achieves this effect by depleting nerves of a pain-mediating neurotransmitter called substance P. Although application of capsaicin cream initially causes a burning feeling, the burning lessens with each application and disappears for most people in a few days. Creams containing 0.025–0.075% of capsaicin are available and may be applied to the affected joints three to five times a day. A doctor should supervise this treatment. Don't use this on irritated or broken skin with a heating pad. Don't touch your eyes after using this material.

Chinese herbs: There have been good studies done in this area. One type of Chinese herb (called by the Un-Chinese name of SKI 306X) is a combination of *Clematis mandshurica, Trichosanthes kirilowii,* and *Prunella vulgaris*. It has been shown to inhibit prostaglandin degradation of cartilage (Choi JH, et al. *Osteoarthritis Cartilage* 2002; 10:471-478).

Curcumin (*Curcuma longa*): This is related to the ginger root and has been shown to block prostaglandin production and stimulate the release of cortisol, which together inhibit inflammation. Curcumin is the active constituent of turmeric, the key ingredient found in many curry dishes, which gives curry its distinct color and flavor. Turmeric has been used in Ayurvedic and Chinese medicine for centuries. Like boswellia, curcumin has also been shown to be effective in the relief of symptoms associated with joint discomfort (based on curcumin's anti-inflammatory and anti-arthritic activity). Clinically, it was found to improve stiffness of joints, morning stiffness, walking time, and joint swelling.

It has been shown to help in two studies involving osteoarthritis and rheumatoid arthritis. (Ammon HP. *Wien Med Wochenschr* 2002; 152 [15-16]:373-8, Amala Cancer Research Centre, Amala Nagar, Trichur. *Indian J Physiol Pharmacol* 1992 Oct;36 [4]:273-5).

Devil's claw (*Harpagophytum procumbens*): Plant used in Africa to treat arthritis. It has anti-inflammatory and analgesic actions. Several open and double-blind trials have been conducted on the anti-arthritic effects of devil's claw (Bone K. *Nutrition and Healing* 1998; October:3;4-8 [review]).The results of these trials have been mixed, so it is unclear whether devil's claw lives up to its reputation in traditional herbal medicine as a remedy for people with rheumatoid arthritis. A typical amount used is 800 mg of encapsulated extracts three times per day or powder in the amount of 4.5–10 grams per day. It appears to reduce pain and inflammation. There is evidence it may have analgesic properties in one osteoarthritis study. It has been touted as a remedy for rheumatoid arthritis. It may allow patients to decrease NSAID dose.

DMSO is a chemical used in wood thinners and solvents. Applied topically, it has been used by veterinarians for years to control inflammation. DMSO (dimethyl sulfoxide) is a colorless, slightly oily liquid that is primarily used as an industrial solvent. The use of DMSO for therapeutic applications is controversial, but some evidence indicates that DMSO has anti-inflammatory properties and alleviates pain when applied to the skin. These effects have been reported particularly with connective tissue diseases such as scleroderma, osteoarthritis, and rheumatoid arthritis and muscle injuries (Jimenez RA, et al. *J Lab Clin Med* 1982; 100:489-500 [review] Swanson BN. *Rev Clin Basic Pharmacol* 1985; 5:1-33, Jacob SW, et al. *Am J Surg* 114:414-26). DMSO applied to the affected area appears to reduce pain by inhibiting transmission of pain messages by nerves. Double-blind and other controlled studies have found a 25 percent DMSO gel effective for pain relief in osteoarthritis of the knee (Eberhardt R, et al. *Fortschritte Med* 1995;113:446-50).

DMSO is an active ingredient in Pennsaid, an anti-inflammatory topical agent for osteoarthritis of the knee. The DMSO helps with absorption through the skin.

Feverfew: Derived from the feverfew plant, it's available as tablets. Animal studies have shown it may reduce pain and inflammation. The active ingredient is parthenolide. Feverfew extracts can reduce swelling and inflammation by inhibiting different substances that are responsible for inflammation such as prostaglandins, leukotrienes, and thromboxane. Phospholipase A is another inflammatory enzyme that appears to be inhibited by feverfew. The anti-inflammatory effect seems to be less than that due to non-steroidal anti-inflammatory drugs (Makheja AM, et al. Lancet 1981; 2:1054-1055, Capasso F Pharm Pharmacol 1986; 38:71-71) .It may cause mouth sores.

Fish oil comes from cold water fish such as mackerel, tuna, halibut, salmon, cod. It contains omega-3 fatty acid (EPA/DHA). Docosahexaenoic acid (DHA), an omega-3 fatty acid, belongs to the class of nutrients called essential fatty acids.

DHA has been shown to reduce levels of blood triglycerides. High triglycerides are linked with heart disease. DHA alone appears to be just as effective as fish oils (which contain both DHA and eicosapentaenoic acid [EPA]) in beneficially lowering triglyceride levels in people at risk for heart disease. In part, this may be because some DHA is converted to EPA in the body. Unlike EPA, however, DHA may not reduce excessive blood clotting (Davidson et al. *J Am Coll Nutr* 1997; 16:236-43; Conquer JA, et al. *J Nutr* 1996;126:3032-9; Nelson GJ, et al. *Lipids* 1997;32:1129-36). DHA supplementation in healthy young men has been shown to decrease the activity of immune cells, such as natural killer (NK) cells and the cells that regulate inflammation responses in the body (Kelley DS, et al. *Lipids* 1999; 34:317-24). The anti-inflammatory effects of DHA may be useful in the management of autoimmune disorders; however, such benefits need to be balanced with the potential for increased risk of infections. In at least 20 clinical trials, it has proven effective in reducing anti-inflammatory drug use (Lau CS, et al. *Br J Rheumatol* 1993; 17:65-71) in rheumatoid arthritis. Either capsules or just plain eating cold water fish will provide this. As mentioned earlier, fish oil can thin the blood so use caution if you are taking blood thinners. As a plus, it lowers triglyceride levels in the blood. While studies have been heavily weighted towards rheumatoid arthritis, there is no reason why it might not work as an anti-inflammatory agent for osteoarthritis as well.

Flaxseed: This contains alpha linoleic acid which is converted to omega -3 oil, a fish oil that reduces inflammation. Like most vegetable oils, flaxseed oil contains linoleic acid, an essential fatty acid needed for survival. But unlike most oils, it also contains significant amounts of another essential fatty acid, alpha linolenic acid (ALA).
ALA is an omega-3 fatty acid. To a limited extent, the body turns ALA into eicosapentaenoic acid (EPA)—an omega-3 fatty acid found in fish oil, which in turn converts to beneficial prostaglandins. (Prostaglandins are hormone-like substances made in many parts of the body rather than coming from one organ, as most hormones do.)

Frankincense: It's also known as Boswellia serrata. Frankincence has been used as a healing herb. It is found primarily in North Africa. This herb may have anti-inflammatory properties and has been used for treatment of arthritis in Middle Eastern culture for centuries. It's been shown to provide relief in both osteoarthritis and rheumatoid arthritis in clinical studies (Chopra A, et al. *Arthritis Rheum* 1996;39:S283; Chopra A, et al. *Arthritis Rheum* 1998;41:S198).

Ginger is another Ayurvedic herb used to treat people with arthritis. A small number of case studies suggest that taking 6 to 50 grams of fresh or powdered ginger per day may reduce the symptoms of rheumatoid arthritis (Srivastava KC, et al. *Med Hypoth* 1992; 39:342-8.) This root is anti-inflammatory and analgesic. It blocks the production of both leukotrienes as well as prostaglandins. One study showed it was effective in patients with osteoarthritis of the knee (Wigler I, et al. *Osteoarthritis Cartilage* 2003; 11:783-789). It can be taken in powder form or as a capsule.

Green-lipped mussel is a New Zealand shellfish, from which an extract has been shown to be useful in the treatment of rheumatoid arthritis and osteoarthritis.

Green-lipped mussel inhibits inflammation in the body. Although inflammation is normal under certain conditions, consistent or excessive inflammation can result in pain and damage to the body, including the joints. The human body makes several chemical mediators of inflammation. Levels of these chemicals in the body may be higher in people with RA who are experiencing symptoms than in symptom-free people with arthritis. Evidence indicates that controlling the production of inflammatory mediators in the body may help improve conditions such as arthritis, asthma, psoriasis, and inflammatory bowel disease (including ulcerative colitis and Crohn's disease), all of which involve elements of inflammation (Gursel T, et al. *Prostaglandins Leukot Essent Fatty Acids* 1997;56:205-7, Henderson WR Jr. *Ann Intern Med* 1994;121:684-97).

Research on green-lipped mussel has focused primarily on osteoarthritis and rheumatoid arthritis. Although some studies have failed to demonstrate a therapeutic benefit of green-lipped mussel in people with arthritis, the outcomes of other studies have been more positive (Gibson RG, et al. *Practitioner* 1980; 224:955-60; Audeval B, et al. *Gaz Med Fr* 1986; 38:111; Caughey DE, et al. *Eur J Rheumatol Inflamm* 1983; 6:197-200).

In one trial, both freeze-dried powder and lipid extract of green-lipped mussel were effective at reducing symptoms in 70 percent of people with osteoarthritis and 76 percent of people with rheumatoid arthritis (Gibson SLM, et al. *Comp Ther Med* 1998; 6:122-6). A similar study of people with either osteoarthritis or rheumatoid arthritis showed green-lipped mussel reduced pain in 50 percent and 67 percent of the patients, respectively, after three months of supplementation (Gibson RG, et al. *Lancet* 1981; 1:439, Whitehouse MW, et al. *Inflam Pharmacol* 1997;5:237-46).

Guggul (*Commiphora mukul*): The guggul tree is native to India. The gum from this tree has anti-inflammatory properties. It may be helpful for arthritis. In a preliminary trial, supplementation with 500 mg of a concentrated extract (3.5 percent guggulsterones) of *Commiphora mukul* (guggul) three times per day for one month resulted in a significant improvement in symptoms in people with osteoarthritis of the knee. Double-blind trials are needed to rule out the possibility of a placebo effect (Singh BB, et al. *Altern Ther Health Med* 2003; 9:74–9).

MSM: Methylsulfonylmethane (MSM) is a naturally occurring, organic, sulfur-containing compound related to another sulfur-containing substance, dimethyl sulfoxide (DMSO). MSM is found in small amounts throughout nature and has been detected in small amounts in the blood and urine of humans (Jacob SW, et al. *Ann N Y Acad Sci.* 1983; 411:13-17).

Animal studies have shown that sulfur from oral supplements of MSM is incorporated into body proteins (Richmond VL. *Life Sci* 1986; 39:263-8). Animal studies have also reported that joints affected by osteoarthritis have lower sulfur content (Rizzo R, et al. *J Exp Zool* 1995; 273:82–6), and mice with arthritis given MSM, experience less joint deterioration (Murav'ev Iuv, et al. *Patol Fiziol Eksp Ter* 1991; 2:37-39).

According to a preliminary report, a double-blind trial in people with OA found that MSM, in the amount of 2,250 mg per day, reduced pain after six weeks (Lawrence RM. *Int J of Anti-Aging Med* 1998; 1:50). A precursor of MSM is formed initially by ocean plankton and released into the atmosphere, where it interacts with ozone and sunlight and returns to earth as MSM in rainfall. MSM can be taken up by plants and incorporated into their structure, but no measurement of the MSM content of foods has been done. Supplements containing MSM are available.

Phellodendron Amurense: Extract from the bark of a Chinese tree. Used in China to help with arthritis. Found in at least one study to have an effect on suppressing cellular immune response (Mori H, *Planta Med.* 1994 60(5):445-9). Western data is sparse.

S-adenosyl methionine (SAMe) possesses anti-inflammatory, pain-relieving, and tissue-healing properties that may help protect the health of joints, though the primary way in which SAMe reduces osteoarthritis symptoms is not known. A very large, though uncontrolled, trial (meaning that there was no comparison with placebo) demonstrated "very good" or "good" clinical effect of SAMe in 71% of over 20,000 OA sufferers (Berger R, et al. *Am J Med* 1987; 83:84-8).

In addition to this preliminary research, many double-blind trials have shown that SAMe reduces pain, stiffness, and swelling better than placebo and equal to drugs such as ibuprofen and naproxen in people with OA (Domljan Z, et al. *Int J Clin Pharmacol Ther Toxicol* 1989; 27:329-33; Vetter G. *Am J Med* 1987;83 (Suppl 5A):78-80; Maccagno A. *Am J Med* 1987;83 (Suppl 5A):72-7; Caruso I, et al. *Am J Med* 1987;83 (Suppl 5A):66-71; Marcolongo R, et al. *Curr Ther Res* 1985; 37:82-94; Glorioso S, et al. *Int J Clin Pharmacol Res* 1985; 5:39-49;

Montrone F, et al. *Clin Rheumatol* 1985; 4:484-5). These double-blind trials all used 1,200 mg of SAMe per day. Lower amounts of oral SAMe have also produced reductions in the severity of OA symptoms in preliminary clinical trials.

A two-year, uncontrolled trial showed significant improvement of symptoms after two weeks at 600 mg SAMe daily, followed by 400 mg daily thereafter (Konig B. *Am J Med* 1987; 83:89-94). This amount was also used in a double-blind trial, but participants first received five days of intravenous SAMe (Bradley JD, et al. *J Rheumatol* 1994; 21:905-11).

A review of the clinical trials on SAMe concluded that its efficacy against osteoarthritis was similar to that of conventional drugs but that patients tolerated it better (Di Padova C. *Am J Med* 1987; 83:60-65). Another study demonstrated that SAMe was as effective as celecoxib (Celebrex) but that the onset of action was slower (Najm WI, et al. *BMC Musculoskeletal Disorders* 2004;26:5)

Stinging nettle: Can be made into a tea or a poultice directly applied to the skin. It has substances that are analgesic and anti-inflammatory and has historically been used for joint pain. Topical application with the intent of causing stings to relieve joint pain has been assessed in preliminary and double-blind trials. The results found intentional nettle stings to be safe and effective for relieving the pain of osteoarthritis. The only reported adverse effect is a sometimes painful rash that lasts

6 to 24 hours (Randall C, et al. *Compl Ther Med* 1999; 7:126-31; Randall C, et al. *J R Soc Med* 2000; 93: 305-9). It is high in vitamin K and may decrease the effectiveness of blood thinners.

White willow bark: The active ingredient is salicin---the same ingredient that makes aspirin effective. It has the same side effects as taking aspirin. Another trial found that 1,360 mg of willow bark extract per day (delivering 240 mg of salicin) was somewhat effective in treating pain associated with knee and/or hip osteoarthritis (Schmid B, et al. *Fact* 1998; 3:186).

Vitamin C. This important vitamin is needed to make collagen. It participates in the process of wound healing by promoting the synthesis of collagen. A high intake of antioxidants, especially vitamin C, may reduce the risk of cartilage loss and slow the progression of osteoarthritis. Participants in the Framingham Osteoarthritis Cohort Study who took higher than average amounts of vitamin C had a threefold decrease in the risk of osteoarthritis (McAlindon TE, et al. Do antioxidant micronutrients protect against the development and progression of knee osteoarthritis? *Arthritis Rheum* 1996;39:648-56). Vitamin C, like vitamin E, also protects and enhances cartilage formation. Guinea pigs with experimental osteoarthritis given 150 mg daily of vitamin C demonstrated significantly less cartilage erosion than animals given only 2-4 mg vitamin C (Schwartz ER. The modulation of osteoarthritic development by vitamins C and E. *Int J Vitam Nutr Res* 1984;26:141-6).

Vitamin D. Scientific studies are beginning to demonstrate that vitamin D can help slow the development of osteoarthritis. Researchers at Boston University Medical Center examined the knees of 556 patients during a two-year period. Those patients who showed progressive knee damage due to osteoarthritis also exhibited lower levels of vitamin D. David Felson, an investigator in the study, noted "A vitamin D deficiency could impair the body's ability to repair the damage that arthritis causes in both bone and cartilage" (Felson D. Relation of dietary intake and serum levels of vitamin D to progression of osteoarthritis of the knee among participants in the Framingham Study. *Ann Int Med* 1996; 125:353).

Other complementary therapies
Acupuncture

According to About.com, in a National Health Interview Survey (in 2002), it was determined that 8.2 million adults in the United States had used acupuncture while 2.1 million had used acupuncture the previous year. Within the past two decades, the popularity of acupuncture has grown.

In 1996, the U.S. Food and Drug Administration approved acupuncture needles for use by licensed acupuncture practitioners. The FDA requires the use of sterile, nontoxic needles, labeled for single use only. In practice, a new set of disposable needles taken from a sealed package should be used for each patient. The treatment sites should be swabbed with alcohol or another disinfecting agent before needles are inserted through the skin. Proper technique minimizes complications. The theory regarding how acupuncture may work is this: Traditional Chinese medicine is based in the belief that disease occurs from an imbalance of yin (a passive principle) and yang (an active principle). The imbalance blocks vital energy along pathways of the body known as meridians. There are 12 main meridians, 8 secondary meridians, and 2000 acupuncture points connecting them on the body. As it applies to Western medicine, some think that acupuncture affects nervous system regulation and painkilling biochemicals.

One of the most convincing studies, entitled, "Effectiveness of acupuncture as adjunctive therapy in osteoarthritis of the knee: a randomized, controlled trial" authored by Berman et al appeared in the journal, Annals of Internal Medicine.

It provided evidence on the efficacy of acupuncture for reducing the pain and dysfunction of osteoarthritis.

The objective was to determine whether acupuncture provided greater pain relief and improved function compared with sham acupuncture or education in patients with osteoarthritis of the knee.

It was designed as a randomized, controlled trial. The setting was two outpatient clinics (an integrative medicine facility and a rheumatology facility) located in academic teaching hospitals and 1 clinical trials facility. 570 patients with osteoarthritis of the knee (mean age [+/- SD], 65.5 +/- 8.4 years) were enrolled. The intervention was 23 true acupuncture sessions over 26 weeks. Controls received 6 two-hour sessions over 12 weeks or 23 sham acupuncture sessions over 26 weeks.

Primary outcomes were changes in the Western Ontario and McMaster Universities Osteoarthritis Index (WOMAC) pain and function scores at 8 and 26 weeks. Secondary outcomes were patient global assessment, 6-minute walk distance, and physical health scores of the 36-Item Short-Form Health Survey (SF-36).

The results showed that the participants in the true acupuncture group experienced greater improvement in WOMAC function scores than the sham acupuncture group but not in WOMAC pain score or the patient global assessment. At 26 weeks, the true acupuncture group experienced significantly greater improvement than the sham group in the WOMAC function, WOMAC pain, and patient global assessment.

There were limitations in that at 26 weeks, 43% of the participants in the education group and 25% in each of the true and sham acupuncture groups were not available for analysis.

The conclusions drawn by the researchers were that acupuncture seemed to provide improvement in function and pain relief as an adjunctive therapy for osteoarthritis of the knee when compared with credible sham acupuncture and education control groups.

Chiropractic (The material for this section comes from the Complementary and Alternative Medicine division of the National Institutes of Health).

Chiropractic is a form of health care that focuses on the relationship between the body's structure, primarily of the spine, and function. Doctors of chiropractic, who are also called chiropractors or chiropractic physicians, use a type of hands-on therapy called manipulation (or adjustment) as their core clinical procedure.

Chiropractic is most often used to treat musculoskeletal conditions---problems with the muscles, joints, bones, and connective tissue such as cartilage, ligaments, and tendons. Chiropractic treatment and conventional medical treatments are about equally helpful for low back conditions.

The risk of experiencing complications from chiropractic adjustment of the low back appears to be very low. However, the risk appears to be higher for adjustment of the neck. It is important to inform all of your health care providers about any treatment that you are using or considering, including chiropractic. This will help each provider make sure that all aspects of your health care are working together.

The underlying concepts of chiropractic can be described as follows: The body has a powerful self-healing ability. The body's structure (primarily that of the spine) and its function are closely related, and this relationship affects health. Chiropractic therapy is given with the goals of normalizing this relationship between structure and function and assisting the body as it heals.

Balneotherapy is an old form of therapy for pain relief for people with arthritis. The word "balneo" comes from the Latin word for bath (balneum). Basically, balneotherapy is the process of bathing in thermal or mineral waters. Sulfur-containing mud baths have been shown to alleviate arthritis symptoms. Hydrotherapy, which can be performed under the guidance of certain physical therapists, is occasionally used interchangeably with the word balneotherapy. The goals of balneotherapy for arthritis include:

- Improving range of joint motion
- Increasing muscle strength
- Eliminating muscle spasm
- Enhancing functional mobility
- Easing pain

Homeopathy (From the University of Maryland Website)

Several studies have shown that homeopathic combinations may be as effective as conventional medications for osteoarthritis. Such remedies include:

- A topical homeopathic gel containing comfrey (*Symphytum officinale*), poison ivy (*Rhus toxicodendron*), and marsh-tea (*Ledum palustre*)
- A combination homeopathic preparation containing *R. toxicodendron.*, *Arnica montana* (arnica), *Solanum dulcamara* (climbing nightshade), *Sanguinarra canadensis* (bloodroot), and Sulphur
- A liquid homeopathic preparation containing *R. toxicodendron*, Causticum (potassium hydrate), and *Lac vaccinum* (cow's milk)

Yoga

Yoga is known for its physical, psychological, emotional, and spiritual pluses. In one clinical trial of hand osteoarthritis, the group practicing yoga showed significantly less pain and improved range of motion compared to those participating in non-yoga stretching and strengthening sessions. Some yoga "asanas" (postures) strengthen the quadriceps and emphasize stretching, both of which help people with knee ostreoarthritis. People with arthritis should begin asanas slowly and they should be performed only after a warm up. Look for a reputable instructor who is knowledgeable about modifying movements for people with arthritis.

Tai Chi is occasionally recommended to help relieve osteoarthritis pain. Clinical studies have found the following benefits of tai chi:

- Improved fitness
- Stronger muscles
- Better flexibility
- Reduced percentage of body fat
- Lowered risk of falls in the elderly

In a clinical trial of people with osteoarthritis of the knee or hip, those who practiced tai chi twice a week for 3 months showed significant improvement compared to those in the control group.

Conventional Therapies

The goals of treatment are to reduce pain, maintain or improve mobility, prevent disability, improve quality of life and maintain independence, control associated medical conditions (called co-morbidities) that may aggravate OA, minimize the risks of therapy, and slow the progression of the disease.

Specific treatment may depend on the area affected. General treatment guidelines include the following:

- **Social support.** Patient/family counseling, as well as support groups, can provide social support. It is imperative that the physician and staff maintain an upbeat and empathetic attitude. Patient rapport is extremely important. A patient should be instructed on life style expectations as well as how best to perform activities of daily living. If they continue to work or have hobbies, an occupational therapist can often provide invaluable advice as to how to continue to stay active and engaged.

- **Education.** Patients may learn about their OA through direct teaching by the physician or clinical nursing staff, or through educational materials such as booklets, pamphlets, videotapes, audiotapes, or CDs. Seminars on selected topics can also be beneficial. The Internet has a number of valuable offerings. (www.arthritis-treatment-and-relief.com, www.arthritistreatmentcenter.com)

- **Mood.** Patients will sometimes be reluctant to voice concerns over their arthritis. They may be depressed or stressed.

- **Other aches and pains.** It is not unusual for patients with osteoarthritis to have musculoskeletal pain due to other conditions. Examples would include tendonitis and bursitis. It is not uncommon for patients with inflammatory erosive osteoarthritis to also have trigger finger. Recent studies have shown that patients with osteoarthritis of the knee will, upon questioning, have pain in multiple other areas.

- **Pain assessment** is important. Not only is it helpful to have a baseline gauge, it is also useful to teach a patient different techniques for coping with the pain. When medications (which will be discussed later) are discussed, patients need to be instructed in dosing, timing, and side effects associated with the treatments.

- **Assistive devices.** Generally, the medical staff, including physical and occupational therapists, provide the smaller assistive devices. For larger items, patients need to see a medical equipment supplier. Examples of assistive devices include splints, braces, walkers, canes, and scooters.

- **Weight control.** Because osteoarthritis tends to affect weight-bearing joints, patients must recognize the importance of weight control. In fact, weight reduction for those who are overweight is as important as medication, if not more important. Dietary consultation is advisable. In addition, exercise is critical to reaching and maintaining an ideal weight.

- **Co-morbid conditions.** Other medical conditions that have an impact on the arthritis or its treatment, must be addressed.

Examples would be obesity, diabetes, heart disease, hypertension, hyperlipidemia, and others.

- **Exercise.** A comprehensive exercise program is critical. Patients should be instructed in strengthening, stretching, and range-of-motion exercises. Unfortunately, once the pain of osteoarthritis begins, it is sometimes difficult to get started on a good exercise program. Non-impact or low-impact forms of exercise such as swimming, riding an exercise bike, or using an elliptical trainer or cross-country ski machine are the best. Enlisting the help of a physical therapist skilled in managing arthritis is advisable.

- In addition, thermal (hot or cold) modalities are sometimes used for symptom control. Patients should try both ice and moist heat, as one may prove more effective in a given patient. For acute pain (pain that is less than 24 hours old), a patient should try ice first. The ice pack should not be applied directly to the skin.

Moist heat can be delivered through the use of commercial heating pads. Or, one simple trick is to put a wet towel inside a sealed plastic bag. Zip the bag shut except for a small opening to allow steam to vent. Microwave the bag with the towel inside on high for 2 minutes. Take the bag and wrap it with a moist towel. This "heating pad" will stay warm for approximately 20 minutes. Be careful, though, for microwaves tend to vary in their heating properties!

Warm baths using medicinal salts are often soothing. An excellent product is the Arthritis Bath Salts available at the Arthritis Treatment Center. (Figure 4)

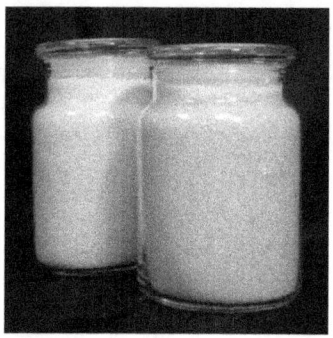

Figure 4

For painful, stiff hands, baths with paraffin (readily available at many discount stores) are very soothing. The paraffin comes in blocks and melts inside the paraffin unit.

Topical agents such as capsaicin cream or Blue Pain Relief may also be beneficial (Figure 5). Blue Pain Relief has the added advantage of containing omega 3 and omega 6 fatty acids, which are anti-inflammatory. Blue Pain Relief is available at the Arthritis Treatment Center.

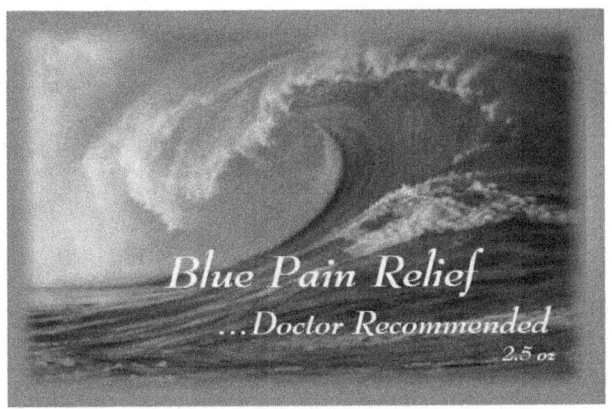

Figure 5

Another topical agent available by prescription is Voltaren gel. This is a topical non-steroidal anti-inflammatory drug. Many people find this treatment very effective. Voltaren gel is indicated for osteoarthritis pain involving the knees and hands. And another new topical anti-inflammatory preparation is Pennsaid. This is applied as drops of diclofenac. Absorption is enhanced by the presence of DMSO. This compound is indicated for osteoarthritis of the knee.

The choice of medication depends on a patient's symptoms!

For very mild pain, some patients require only acetaminophen (Tylenol) or perhaps over-the-counter anti-inflammatory doses of ibuprofen (Advil, Nuprin) or naproxyn (Aleve). For more severe discomfort, a prescription non-steroidal anti-inflammatory drug (NSAID) may be necessary.

Non-steroidal anti-inflammatory drugs are commonly used to treat arthritis because of their analgesic (pain-killing), anti-inflammatory, and antipyretic (fever-reducing) properties. They are also attractive because they lead to rapid pain relief, improved function, lack the central nervous system effects of opioid pain killers, and come in many varieties.

There are two types of cyclooxygenase. Cyclooxygenase 1 (COX-1) produces prostaglandins that are important for normal physiologic function, including protection of the stomach lining, kidney function, platelet function, and maintenance of blood vessels.

Cyclooxygenase 2 (COX-2) produces prostaglandins that are important in the events that cause inflammation. These prostaglandins are localized to inflammatory sites such as inflamed tissue or inflamed joints.

In summary...prostaglandins, which are inhibited by NSAIDs, function in the body to protect the stomach lining, promote clotting of the blood, regulate salt and fluid balance, and maintain blood flow to the kidneys when kidney function is reduced. By decreasing prostaglandins, NSAIDs can cause stomach irritation, bleeding, fluid retention, and decreased kidney function.

Bottom line: NSAIDs work because they block cyclooxygenase and therefore inhibit prostaglandin production.

This mechanism may relate to the variation in response to NSAIDS between patients. Scientific studies have shown a correlation between concentration of the drug and effect, but do not explain the differences in individual patient responses. It is thought that the pharmacokinetic (process by which a drug is absorbed, distributed, metabolized, and eliminated) differences among the various NSAIDs may account for the variability in response. Also entering into the equation are variations in disease, differences in the incidences of side effects, and possibly patient preference for one NSAID over another.

Non-steroidal anti-inflammatory drugs (NSAIDs) are prescribed for a variety of painful conditions, including arthritis, bursitis, tendonitis, gout, menstrual cramps, sprains, strains, and other injuries.

Non-steroidal anti-inflammatory drugs relieve pain, stiffness, swelling, and inflammation, but they do not cure the diseases or injuries responsible for these problems. Some non-steroidal anti-inflammatory drugs can be bought over the counter; others are available only with a prescription from a physician or dentist.

Among the drugs in this group are piroxicam (Feldene), meclofenamate sodium (Meclomen), sulindac (Clinoril), tolmetin sodium (Tolectin), ketoprofen (Orudis), diclofenac (Voltaren), etodolac (Lodine), flurbiprofen (Ansaid), ibuprofen (Motrin, Advil, Rufen), ketorolac (Toradol), nabumetone (Relafen), naproxen

(Naprosyn); naproxen sodium (Aleve, Anaprox, Naprelan); oxaprozin (Daypro) and meloxicam (Mobic). They are sold as tablets, capsules, caplets, liquids, and rectal suppositories, and some are available in chewable, extended-release, or delayed-release forms.

Recommended doses vary, depending on the patient, the type of non-steroidal anti-inflammatory drug prescribed, the condition for which the drug is prescribed, and the form in which it is used. Patients should always take non-steroidal anti-inflammatory drugs exactly as directed. If using nonprescription (over-the-counter) types, follow the directions on the package label. For prescription types, check with the physician who prescribed the medicine or the pharmacist who filled the prescription. Don't be afraid of asking questions! Never take larger or more frequent doses, and do not take the drug for longer than directed. Patients who take non-steroidal anti-inflammatory drugs for severe arthritis must take them regularly over a long time. The reason is that anti-inflammatory effect is seen only when the drugs reach a certain serum level...and that requires constant dosing. These drugs do have analgesic effects when taken sporadically, but this is insufficient to treat the inflammation of arthritis. Several weeks may be needed to feel the results, so it is important to keep taking the medicine, even if it does not seem to be working at first.

When taking non-steroidal anti-inflammatory drugs in tablet, capsule, or caplet form, you should always take them with a full, eight-ounce glass of water or milk. Taking these drugs with food or an antacid may help prevent stomach irritation.

Non-steroidal anti-inflammatory drugs can cause a number of side effects, some of which may be very serious.

Side effects that occur most frequently are heartburn and prevention of normal platelet stickiness, which can lead to prolonged bleeding. Next most common are stomach or small bowel bleeding, ulceration, or even bowel perforation.

The really frightening aspect of NSAID therapy is that up to 91 percent of patients who eventually have abnormal findings at the time of endoscopy (looking inside the stomach with a special telescope), report no symptoms (Larkai EN, et al., Am J Gastroenterol 1987; 82: 1153-1158).

Less commonly, patients can develop central nervous system side effects, liver toxicity, rashes, kidney damage, which may or may not be reversible, and lung problems. These side effects are more likely when the drugs are taken in large doses, or for a long time, or when two or more non-steroidal anti-inflammatory drugs are taken together. And older patients are often taking aspirin for heart prophylaxis already!!

Rheumatologists can help patients weigh the risks and benefits of taking these medicines for long periods.

So what is the <u>real</u> magnitude of the problem associated with NSAID use?

- More than 100 million prescriptions for NSAIDs are written each year
- NSAIDs are prescribed in half of all office visits for arthritis.
- NSAIDs are dispensed to more than 14 million arthritis patients.
- Damage to the stomach lining is visible in 20-40 percent of users.
- NSAID users account for 15-60 percent of hospital admissions for GI bleeding.

Mortality (the risk of dying) from a gastrointestinal complication related to NSAIDs is third only to cigarette smoking and motor vehicle accidents!

NSAIDs lead to more than 100,000 hospitalizations a year and 10,000 to 20,000 deaths/ year. In fact, of the total treatment cost related to arthritis care, about 1/3 of the cost relates to treatment of adverse GI effects from NSAIDs!

The most common side effects are stomach pain or cramps, nausea, vomiting, indigestion, diarrhea, heartburn, headache, dizziness or lightheadedness, and drowsiness. The unfortunate problem is that severe gastrointestinal problems can develop without prior symptoms!

People at most risk for NSAID gastropathy (the syndrome that describes the side effects that anti-inflammatory drugs cause on the gut) are:

- 60 years of age
- smokers
- prior history of ulcer or gastrointestinal bleed
- arthritis-related disability
- high dose or multiple NSAIDs
- concurrent prednisone use
- history of cardiovascular disease
- concurrent use of antacids

Also, it appears that patients who have Helicobacter pylori, the bacteria that causes routine peptic ulcer disease, have a higher risk of getting ulcers than patients who do not. So the risk of getting ulcers is actually multiplied when a patient who has H. pylori is placed on NSAIDs.

As mentioned earlier, patients on NSAIDs can develop small bowel problems, and patients with a history of inflammatory bowel disease can have a flare of their disease as a result of NSAIDs. Protection of the stomach can be accomplished with a number of different medicines. The best so far appear to be what are called the proton pump inhibitors.

A study in the United Kingdom revealed ibuprofen as the lowest risk for causing serious upper gastrointestinal distress. Naproxen, indomethacin, and diclofenac were viewed as an intermediate risk. Azapropazone and piroxicam had the highest risk.

Severe liver disease, including abnormal elevations of liver function tests and hepatitis, also can occur as a result of NSAIDS.

Do not take acetaminophen, aspirin, or other salicylates along with other non-steroidal anti-inflammatory drugs for more than a few days unless directed to do so by a physician.

Some non-steroidal anti-inflammatory drugs can increase the chance of bleeding after surgery (including dental surgery), so anyone who is taking the drugs should alert the physician or dentist before surgery. Avoiding the medicine or switching to another type in the days prior to surgery may be necessary.

Some people feel drowsy, dizzy, confused, lightheaded, or less alert when using these drugs. Blurred vision or other vision problems also are possible side effects. For these reasons, anyone who takes these drugs should not drive, use machines or do anything else that might be dangerous until they have found out how the drugs affect them.

Non-steroidal anti-inflammatory drugs make some people more sensitive to sunlight. Even brief exposure to sunlight can cause severe sunburn, rashes, redness, itching, blisters, or discoloration. In rare instances, NSAIDs have caused a life-threatening condition called Stevens-Johnson syndrome. Here the patient loses their skin. It's like a total body third-degree burn! Vision changes also may occur. To reduce the chance of these problems, avoid direct sunlight, especially from mid-morning to mid-afternoon; wear protective clothing, a hat, and sunglasses; and use a sunscreen with a skin protection factor (SPF) rating of at least 15, and preferably higher. Do not use sunlamps, tanning booths or tanning beds while taking these drugs.

People with certain medical conditions and people who are taking some other medicines can have problems if they take non-steroidal anti-inflammatory drugs. Before taking these drugs, be sure to let the physician know about any of these conditions:

Let the physician know about any allergies to foods, dyes (especially tartrazine---a commonly used yellow food dye), preservatives, or other substances. Anyone who has had reactions to non-steroidal anti-inflammatory drugs in the past should also check with a physician before taking them again. NSAID allergy can be life-threatening due to the possibility of anaphylactic shock. Aspirin has caused the heart to stop completely!

Women who are pregnant or who plan to become pregnant should check with their physicians before taking these medicines. Whether non-steroidal anti-inflammatory drugs cause birth defects in people is unknown, but some do cause birth defects in laboratory animals. If taken late in pregnancy, these drugs may prolong pregnancy, lengthen labor time, cause problems during delivery, or affect the heart or blood flow of the fetus.

Some non-steroidal anti-inflammatory drugs pass into breast milk. Women who are breastfeeding should check with their physicians before taking these drugs.

A number of medical conditions may influence the effects of non-steroidal anti-inflammatory drugs. Anyone who has any of the conditions listed below should tell his or her physician about the condition before taking non-steroidal anti-inflammatory drugs:

- Stomach or intestinal problems like inflammatory bowel disease---ulcerative colitis or Crohn's disease.
- Liver disease
- Kidney disease, including kidney stones
- Heart disease
- Hypertension
- Blood disorders such as low platelet counts, low white blood cell counts, or severe anemia
- Bleeding problems
- Diabetes mellitus

- Hemorrhoids or rectal bleeding
- Asthma
- Parkinson's disease
- Seizure disorders
- Fluid retention
- Alcohol abuse

People who have mouth sores should tell the physician about them before starting to take non-steroidal anti-inflammatory drugs. Sores or ulcers that appear in the mouth while taking the drug can be a sign of serious side effects. This may be an indication that a serious condition called Stevens-Johnson syndrome is occurring. Stevens-Johnson is life-threatening!

Some non-steroidal anti-inflammatory drugs contain sugar or sodium, so anyone on a low-sugar or low-sodium diet should be sure to tell his or her physician.

Cigarette smokers may be more likely to have unwanted side effects from this medicine.

Taking non-steroidal anti-inflammatory drugs with certain other drugs may affect the way the drugs work or increase the risk of unwanted side effects.

The effectiveness of anti-hypertensive drugs may be compromised by the use of NSAIDs.

Rarely, neurologic complications such as meningitis, psychosis, and thinking problems have been reported. On the flip side, there is some evidence that NSAIDs may help to forestall Alzheimer's disease. Much has been written, and with good reason, about the effects of NSAIDs on kidney function. These drugs can cause kidney damage consisting of damage to the kidney itself as well as abnormalities of kidney function resulting in abnormal retention of fluid.

Serious side effects are rare, but sometimes do occur. If any of the following side effects occur, stop taking the medicine and get emergency medical care as soon as possible:

- Facial swelling
- Swelling of the legs or arms
- Rapid weight gain
- Fainting or seizures
- Shortness of breath
- Irregular heart rate
- Chest tightness/ pain
- Abdominal cramps or burning
- Fever
- Nausea, heartburn, or indigestion
- Mouth ulcers/sores

- Rashes
- Bleeding, eg. nosebleeds, vomiting blood
- Tarry black stool
- Excessive bruising
- Severe headaches
- taste

Aspirin-sensitive asthma is a serious side-effect occurring in about 2-6% of asthmatic patients. This association is strongest in patients who also have nasal polyps.

A number of less common, temporary side effects are also possible. They usually do not need medical attention and will disappear once the body adjusts to the medicine. If they continue or interfere with normal activity, check with the physician. Among these side effects are:

- Constipation, gas, bloating
- Change in teaste
- Sweating
- Restlessness, anxiety
- Drowsiness

Non-steroidal anti-inflammatory drugs may interact with a variety of other medicines. When this happens, the effects of the drugs may change, and the risk of side effects may be greater. Anyone who takes these drugs should let the physician know all other medicines he or she is taking. Among the drugs that may interact with non-steroidal anti-inflammatory drugs are:

- Blood thinners like warfarin (Coumadin)
- Other non-steroidal anti-inflammatory drugs
- Heparin
- Tetracycline
- Cyclosporine
- Heart drugs like digitalis (Digoxin)
- Lithium
- Anti-seizure drugs like phenytoin (Dilantin)
- Zidovudine (AZT, Retrovir)

Pain and inflammation sometime occur in a circadian rhythm (daily rhythmic cycle based on a 24 hour interval).

Therefore, NSAIDs may be more effective at certain times. If you're having more pain and stiffness in the morning, it may be advisable to take your NSAID in the evening.

NSAIDs are divided into two groups: those with plasma (blood) half-lives less than six hours (i.e. aspirin, diclofenac, ibuprofen) and those with half-lives greater than ten hours (i.e. diflunisal, piroxicam, and sulindac). Since it takes three to five half-lives to stabilize blood levels, NSAIDs with longer half-lives sometimes are more effective when a loading dose is given (large dose given initially). The "half-life" is the time it takes a drug to go down to half of its initial level.

Synovial fluid (joint fluid) concentrations are roughly 60 percent of plasma concentrations regardless of type of NSAID or its half-life. Synovial fluid is the site of action of NSAIDs.

NSAIDs are 95 percent albumin (protein) bound. The unbound fraction of the NSAID is increased in patients with low albumin concentrations such as in active rheumatoid arthritis and the elderly. What this means is that more drug is available for both effects, as well as side-effects!

Since NSAIDs bind to plasma proteins, they may be displaced by or may displace other plasma-bound drugs such as coumadin, methotrexate, digoxin, cyclosporine, oral antidiabetic agents, and sulfa drugs. This interaction can increase either therapeutic or toxic effects of either drug.

Due to their different chemical properties, some NSAIDs have substantial biliary (bile ducts, gallbladder) excretion (i.e., indomethacin, sulindac), and others are metabolized pre-excretion, while a few are sent out in the urine unchanged.

NSAID studies have shown a variation in patient response attributed to a lower rate of sticking with one NSAID when other NSAIDs are known to be available. Patients want a drug they think will be better for them. Whether it's a drug their neighbor's on, or one they saw on T.V., or whatever...The response to and preference of an NSAID may relate to more than just symptom control.

About 60 percent of patients will respond to any single NSAID.

A trial period of two weeks should be given for anti-inflammatory effectiveness to be observed.

Antipyretic and anti-inflammatory effects of NSAIDs can mask the signs and symptoms of infection.

Long-term use of NSAIDs may have a damaging effect on chondrocyte (cartilage) function.

So what are a few don'ts?

- Don't take another person's NSAID.
- Don't alter the dose of your NSAID without talking to the doctor.
- Don't operate machinery or drive until you know your NSAID won't make you drowsy.

- Don't take your NSAID with coffee, alcohol, or anything else that might upset your stomach.
- Don't combine NSAIDS without talking to your doctor.
- If you're going to have surgery, you will need to stop your NSAID about seven to ten days before surgery.

The theory behind the Cox-2 selective NSAIDs (celecoxib [Celebrex]), is that by blocking cyclo-oxygenase-2, the enzyme responsible for inflammation, and sparing cyclo-oxygenase-1, there should be just as much relief of inflammation with fewer complications due to ulcers.

And for the most part, that is true. These drugs confer a measure of safety compared with the older agents. Unfortunately, there are problems. For instance, patients who take aspirin for cardiac prophylaxis have a risk of gastrointestinal problems that is not a whole lot different from patients taking traditional NSAIDs. The weight of current evidence suggests that patients taking either traditional NSAIDs or COX-2s who are at increased risk for cardiovascular disease should take anti-platelet drugs (i.e., aspirin) if there is no reason not to. There is an increased risk of cardiovascular events with all NSAIDs regardless if they are COX-2 selective drugs or not. The risk is the same.

NSAIDs and COX-2 inhibitors should be used with caution in patients with a history of congestive heart failure or who have kidney problems, diabetes, or dehydration.

And patients with a history of sulfa allergy should avoid celecoxib. There is some evidence (Stevenson, et al., J Allergy Clin Immunol. 2001; 108:47-53) that COX-2 drugs can be used in patients with aspirin-sensitive asthma. Be careful!!

And while NSAIDs don't really have disease-modifying effects per se, they are an important part of therapy because they do provide the symptom relief, which is so important in the management of the patient with arthritis.

Some experts advocate the use of drugs called proton pump inhibitors (Protonix, Prilosec, Nexium) in conjunction with NSAIDS to help counteract the possibility of gastrointestinal complications.

A newer anti-inflammatory medicine, Vimovo, combines the anti-inflammatory effects of naproxyn with the stomach protecting properties of a proton pump inhibitor.

Another anti-inflammatory option is Celebrex, a non-steroidal anti-inflammatory drug which is a COX-2 inhibitor. That means it has less effect on the protective lining of the stomach than other non COX-2 inhibitors.

Celebrex should not be used in patients who are allergic to sulfa. It can be used effectively in patient who must take low dose aspirin for heart and stroke prophylaxis because it does not interfere with the action of aspirin, while the other NSAIDS do.

All non-steroidal anti-inflammatory drugs, whether they are COX-2 selective or not, have an increased risk of cardiovascular events such as heart attack and stroke associated with them.

Some patients with severe pain may need supplemental analgesic medication along with their NSAID. Tramadol (Ultram) can be used. Side-effects include nausea, dizziness, headache, and, rarely, seizures in patients also taking selective serotonin reuptake inhibitors. Narcotic analgesics such as codeine, and even oxycodone may be required in severe cases. Propoxyphene is an analgesic which, while effective, was removed from the market by the FDA in November 2010 because of concerns related to an increased risk of heart rhythm abnormalities. Non-steroidal anti-inflammatory drugs can be combined with analgesics if necessary.

Patients with severe osteoarthritis often are treated with intra-articular (into the joint) injections of steroid. The theory is that local inflammation will be suppressed and pain will be relieved. For the most part, this is true. However, if the OA is very advanced, the benefit of steroid injection will be short-lived.

Guidelines for the treatment of knee osteoarthritis were outlined by a task force for the European League Against Rheumatism (EULAR) Standing Committee for Clinical Trials. The taskforce recommended intra-articular steroid injection for acute exacerbation of knee pain. This task force performed an evidence-based review and concluded at least 1 randomized control trial recommended intra-articular steroid for patients with osteoarthritis. It was noted that intra-articular steroid injections were effective for only short-term pain relief and that there are no predictors of success of treatment, such as the presence or absence of such factors as joint effusion (fluid within the joint), degree of x-ray change, age, or obesity.

The American College of Rheumatology Subcommittee on Osteoarthritis Guidelines developed both non-pharmacological and pharmacological recommendations for the treatment of osteoarthritis of the knee. These recommendations include: use of intra-articular steroid injection for patients with acute exacerbations who had evidence for joint inflammation, and joint aspiration accompanying the intra-articular injection for "short-term relief."

There is very little question that in patients for whom joint inflammation is a significant problem (e.g., in the hip, knee, finger, ankle, toe), steroid injection may help. Steroid injections are a mixed blessing, however. Although they are helpful for symptom control, it is difficult to predict the length of time that a single injection will be effective. Also, there is evidence that steroids injected into joints can actually lead to more cartilage deterioration. Finally, steroids should not be injected into an individual joint more than three times per year. It is imperative that diagnostic ultrasound be used to ensure proper placement of the injecting needle.

For patients who do not respond to oral medications and steroid injections, another option may be visco-supplementation. The normal knee joint produces synovial fluid, a thick slippery substance that nourishes cartilage and allows smooth gliding of the cartilage surfaces. With arthritis, the amount of synovial fluid made by the joint is reduced.

In instances when other therapies do not provide the desired relief, viscosupplements are sometimes used. These are gel-like substances (hyaluronates) that mimic the properties of naturally occurring joint fluid.

These hyaluronates actually supplement the viscous properties of synovial fluid. Injection of hyaluronates is done using either fluoroscopic or ultrasound needle guidance. Currently, hyaluronate injections are approved for the treatment of osteoarthritis of the knee in those who have failed to respond to more conservative therapy. The number of injections performed varies with the type of viscosupplement used. There are some preparations where only one injection is required. Others require five for the best response.

Currently, there are five FDA approved hyaluronates:

- Hyalgan
- Synvisc
- Euflexa
- Supartz
- Orthovisc

We have found Synvisc to be the least well tolerated viscosupplement because of pseudoseptic reactions. These are reactions some people get after an injection that can look like a joint infection. There is marked swelling, redness, and heat and some patients can develop a mild fever. Other viscosupplements appear to be better tolerated. Many physicians have found viscosupplements to be effective. Some investigators have claimed that viscosupplements may have disease-modifying effects. As with steroid injections, ultrasound guidance is highly recommended in order to ensure accuracy.

While a few studies have suggested that the benefit derived from visco-supplementation is modest, we have found these preparations to be very helpful. Visco-supplementation is most commonly used in the knee. However, it may be used in other joints, including the hip, shoulder, ankle, toe, and base of the thumb. Examples of visco-supplements are Hyalgan, Synvisc, Euflexa, and Supartz. In our clinic, we use Supartz because it seems to get the best results. Also, the chance of severe flare-ups in arthritis is much lower with Supartz and

Hyalgan than with the other visco-supplements, particularly Synvisc which has been associated with inflammatory flares after injection.

Case history: A 65-year-old executive came to our clinic to find out what could be done for his knees. He had played football at a Big 10 university, but had not suffered severe injuries in college. For the past year, he had experienced increasing stiffness, pain, and swelling in his knees. Clinical examination showed evidence of osteoarthritis. Knee x-ray films confirmed this. He underwent arthroscopic debridement, visco-supplementation, and bracing of his right knee (Figure 6). He also began taking glucosamine and chondroitin (Joint Food; Figure 4-7). At 1 year after treatment, he is doing well.

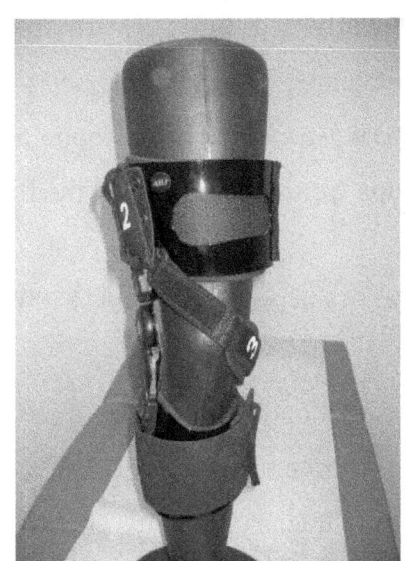

Figure 6 - Brace for patients with osteoarthritis of the knee. This actually reduces the amount of weight on the side of the knee that is affected by osteoarthritis.

European studies indicate that glucosamine and chondroitin sulfate are effective for symptom control; they also show these compounds may have disease-modifying properties.

The recent GAIT (Glucosamine in Arthritis Intervention Trial) study (Clegg D, et al. Glucosamine, Chondroitin Sulfate, and the two in combination for painful knee osteoarthritis. New Engl J Med. 2006;354:795-808) was the first and largest study of glucosamine and chondroitin in the United States.

A total of 1,583 people participated in the study. People age 40 or older with knee pain and documented x-ray evidence of osteoarthritis were eligible to participate. Participants could not have used glucosamine for 3 months and chondroitin sulfate for 6 months prior to entering the study. Participants were about 59 years of age, on average, and nearly two-thirds of participants were women. Of the 1,583 study participants, 78 percent (1,229) were in the mild pain subgroup and 22 percent (354) were in the moderate-to-severe pain subgroup. The groups were randomized to the following treatment groups:

- Glucosamine alone: 1500 mg daily given as 500 mg three times a day
- Chondroitin sulfate alone: 1200 mg daily given as 400 mg three times a day
- Glucosamine plus chondroitin sulfate combined: same doses- 1500 mg and 1200 mg daily

- Celecoxib: 200 mg daily
- Acetaminophen: participants were allowed to take up to 4000 mg (500 mg tablets) per day to control pain, except for the 24 hours before pain was assessed.

The results were the following:

- Participants taking the positive control, celecoxib, experienced statistically significant pain relief versus placebo--about 70 percent of those taking celecoxib had a 20 percent or greater reduction in pain versus about 60 percent for placebo.
- Overall, there were no significant differences between the other treatments tested and placebo.
- For a subset of participants with moderate-to-severe pain, glucosamine combined with chondroitin sulfate provided statistically significant pain relief compared to placebo--about 79 percent had a 20 percent or greater reduction in pain versus about 54 percent for placebo. According to the researchers, because of the small size of this subgroup these findings should be considered preliminary and need to be confirmed in further studies.
- For participants in the mild pain subset, glucosamine and chondroitin sulfate together or alone did not provide statistically significant pain relief.

The results of this study have been scrutinized and argued about. Our take on this is that the combination does work but there are caveats. The glucosamine preparation in the GAIT trial was glucosamine hydrochloride and not glucosamine sulfate. We recommend the sulfate. Also, the moderate to severe group did improve and that is noteworthy.

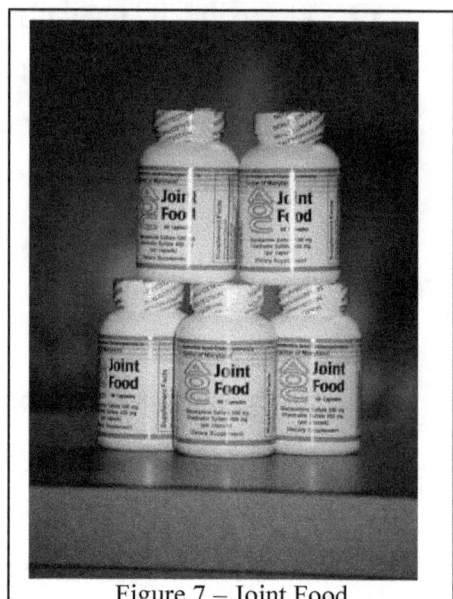

Figure 7 – Joint Food

We feel it is critical to make sure that the preparation used is pure. In the United States, nutritional supplements are not regulated, and the quality and content of these preparations vary a great deal. In Europe, however, glucosamine and chondroitin are highly regulated for content and purity. Therefore, it is important to use a preparation made according to European standards of purity, such as Joint Food (Figure 7).

The preparation taken for osteoarthritis should contain glucosamine sulfate as glucosamine sulfate 2 KCl, 500 mg, and chondroitin sulfate, 400 mg. So patients take 1,500 mg of glucosamine and 1,200 mg of chondroitin if they take the recommended dosage of three capsules a day. Glucosamine is also available as a hydrochloride, but fewer studies have been done with this form. Generally, it takes approximately 2 months to notice a difference.

Glucosamine/chondroitin compounds are relatively safe. Some people have reported mild side-effects, such as increased gas or loose stools. Theoretical concerns regarding their use in patients with severe diabetes have been mentioned, but we have not found this to be a problem. Patients with sulfa allergies may be able to take the pure forms of glucosamine/chondroitin. It may be wise for patients on blood-thinning medications to have more frequent coagulation laboratory tests when they start to take glucosamine/chondroitin—just to be safe. Those who are allergic to shellfish should exercise caution, but most people can take these supplements.

Disease-modifying drugs

Unfortunately, the number of disease-modifying medications available for osteoarthritis is rather limited. Some physicians use hydroxychloroquine (Plaquenil), an antimalarial drug that is sometimes used for rheumatoid arthritis. There have also been reports that minocycline or doxycycline may be effective in patients with OA.

In some patients whose OA has a severe erosive inflammatory component, we have used methotrexate and prednisone with good results. These patients have a disease that is a close cousin to rheumatoid arthritis. Interleukin 1, a pro-inflammatory cytokine, may play a big role in OA.

Other remedies…

Braces that unload the narrowed compartment in the knee may often alleviate symptoms (Figure 6). These braces work by actually reducing the amount of pressure that is placed on the narrowed part of the joint. Many patients find these braces to be helpful.

Another type of treatment is the transcutaneous electrical stimulator- or TENS unit. This is a device that transmits a small electric current to the affected area. By blocking the transmission of pain impulses in the skin, patients sometimes get relief from the pain of osteoarthritis.

Along the same line, some people have begun to use a new type of treatment called electrobiologic therapy. The Food and Drug Administration (FDA) approved the use of one home device, the Bionicare BIO-1000 System, "for use as adjunctive therapy in reducing the level of pain and symptoms associated with osteoarthritis of the knee and for overall improvement of the knee as assessed by the physician's global evaluation." Patients place electrodes on their knee and apply a low-amplitude electrical stimulation (Figure 8). The theory is that the electrical stimulation helps cartilage cells to regenerate. Some studies have demonstrated improved mobility, as well as improved joint function. Patients must wear the Bionicare device for 6 to 10 hours per day. Improvement usually occurs within 2 to 4 weeks. Effects are similar to those of NSAIDs as far as pain relief.

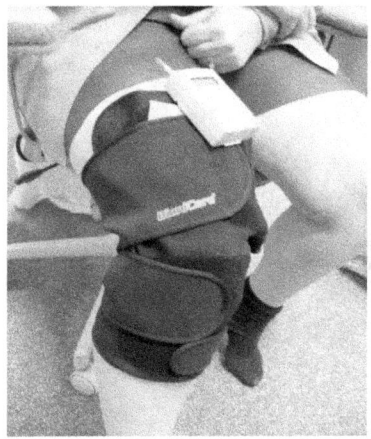

Bionicare Electrotherapy device
This is worn as a wrap around the knee usually at night. Patients adjust the amount of electrical stimulation.

Figure 8

This device has been upgraded so that it is now used in conjunction with an unloading type knee brace.

Here is an excerpt from their website…

The OActive osteoarthritis knee brace is a low profile unloading brace with adjustable

Correction (Figure 9). The BioniCare technology employs an electrical stimulation system that was cleared for marketing by the FDA in 2003, and indicated for use as "an adjunctive therapy for relieving pain and symptoms associated with osteoarthritis of the knee and for overall improvement of the knee as assessed by the physician's global assessment.

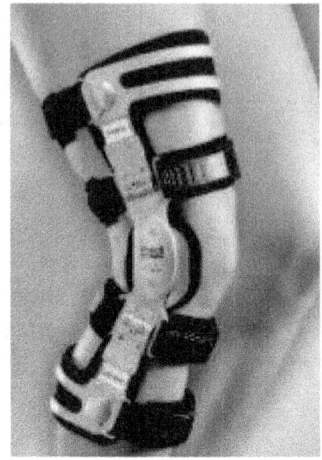

Figure 9

In patients who have received no relief from all these other remedies, more aggressive procedures should be considered. Arthroscopic joint debridement has fallen out of favor as a treatment largely based on the findings of a negative article in the *New England Journal of Medicine* in 2002 (Moseley JB, O'MalleyK, Petersen NJ, Menke TJ,et al. A Controlled Trial of Arthroscopic Surgery for Osteoarthritis of the Knee. New Engl J Med. 2002; 347:81-88). However, it should still be considered for those patients who have intractable knee pain as a result of osteoarthritis, particularly if there is evidence of tearing of the meniscus.

Arthroscopic debridement for other joints may be undertaken on a case by case evaluation. (Arthroscopy is also done for the hip joint at some centers.) Patient selection is critical. This procedure is not effective for patients who are tremendously obese, who have severe OA, or who have no signs of inflammation. It is a reasonable alternative for patients who fit the right criteria, however.

We published a paper outlining our early experience with arthroscopic treatment of OA involving the base of the thumb. (Wei, N, Delauter, SK, Beard, S. Arthroscopic Debridement and Viscosupplementation: A Minimally Invasive Treatment for Symptomatic Osteoarthritis Involving the Base of the Thumb. J Clin Rheum. 2002; 8 (3):125-129). We combined an arthroscopy procedure with an injection of Hyalgan. This procedure has helped a number of patients who otherwise would have required a much more extensive open procedure.

One type of treatment that has been evaluated in uncontrolled trials is prolotherapy. This is the injection of a solution such as dextrose or sodium morhuate. These compounds cause a local inflammatory response and may stimulate cartilage repair. The lack of controlled trials leaves this type of treatment suspect.

Other uncontrolled studies have mentioned the use of platelet-rich plasma (PRP). One study from the Orthohealing Center in Los Angeles described a series of fourteen patients with osteoarthritis of the knee who responded to this therapy. The theory is a good one since PRP also stimulates an acute inflammatory response which should stimulate cartilage repair. Unfortunately, again, without the presence of well-controlled studies, it's difficult to know if this substance really is as effective as claimed.

For patients with severe OA, a number of surgical solutions are available. In patients who have a relatively localized defect, who are young, and who are otherwise in good health, two types of cartilage transplant are possible. The first is osteochondral grafting—inserting a cartilage plug obtained from a non-weight-bearing area of the knee into the weight-bearing defect. In the second type of transplant, autologous chondrocyte implantation, cartilage cells are harvested from a non-weight-bearing area of the knee, grown outside the body using tissue culture techniques, and re-implanted into the cartilage defect. The defect is then covered with a thin protective membrane. This technique requires at least two surgical procedures and a 6-month period of non-weight-bearing after the chondrocytes are put in place…not a procedure to be taken lightly!

For patients who have cartilage loss in one compartment, osteotomy can be helpful. This is a procedure in which a wedge of bone is removed from the shin bone. This removal allows the knee to line up in a way that improves the distribution of the mechanical forces.

Sometimes, patients find the use of heel wedges in the shoes helpful in correcting the knee misalignment. Obviously, heel wedges should be tried before surgery.

Surgery

(This material is taken from the National Institutes of Health Osteoarthritis Fact Sheet)

Development of longer-lasting materials and design of artificial joints that more closely mimic the natural movement of the knee are making total knee replacements more popular and better suited for younger, more active patients who have osteoarthritis.

Joint replacement involves removing the cartilage from either side of the joint and putting metal and plastic in its place. A joint replacement is called a "prosthesis." New materials and new surgical techniques for joint replacement have been developed over the years. A prosthesis can be cemented or non-cemented. Usually, a cemented prosthesis is used in older people. The non-cemented version is better for younger, active people. An important point: good bone quality is required so bone can grow into the prosthesis to keep it tight and secure.

Joint prostheses are typically composed of titanium and cobalt chrome. Tantalum, a porous metal, is being used more frequently now.

A joint prosthesis is expected to last about 10 to 15 years, which depends on the age of the patient. The problem here is that a revision- a second, third, and possibly fourth procedure are required to replace the worn out prosthesis in patients who get joint replacement at a young age.

In 2006, approximately 542,000 total knee replacement surgeries were performed in the United States. Surgical advances have made hip replacements safer for older patients, many of whom have other conditions that previously would have made them ineligible for the procedure. Of the approximately 254,000 hip replacement surgeries performed in the United States in 2000, almost half were in patients over 75 years of age. If a person needs two knee replacement surgeries because of severe arthritis in each leg, replacing both joints at the same time is no more risky than spacing the procedures so the patient can recover between the first and second operations. The development of less-invasive surgical approaches and preoperative regimens has led to decreased hospital stays and recovery time. For example, NIH researchers demonstrated that osteoarthritis patients who participated in an exercise program before receiving an artificial knee or hip were more likely to return home instead of going to an inpatient rehabilitation facility immediately after leaving the hospital, a finding that is likely to have profound cost-savings if widely adopted.

Knee replacements can either be partial or total depending on the situation.

Up until about five years ago, it was not uncommon to see women with knee replacements that were still causing pain. The reason?

Some of these replacements were originally designed for men so they didn't really fit right and caused irritation of the peroneal nerve, which caused pain. We've been able to help control the pain in our patients by administering ultrasound guided peroneal nerve hydrodissection to free up the trapped nerve. This procedure can be repeated.

However, the more important development is the realization that this was a real problem and now women are being fit with "female" type replacements.

C'mon, Dr. Wei...is that all you have for OA?

Yes, it's true. Ironic as it is, there are fewer effective treatments available for OA, which affects approximately 50 million people in the United States, than there are for rheumatoid arthritis, which affects roughly 2 million people in the United States. Why is that?

Well, for one reason, autoimmune diseases have been a "sexier" disease to study in the laboratory. And up until the last 15 to 20 years, most rheumatologists were academic physicians who spent a lot of time in the laboratory doing basic research. For another reason, the area of cartilage biology was not considered very progressive for many years. Now, though, it seems that OA is drawing more interest.

A recent study reported the effectiveness of leeches (yeah...those leeches!) for the treatment of OA of the knee. Hirudin, a bioactive substance in leech saliva, may be the reason why patients improved. Hirudin apparently has anti-inflammatory properties.

We recently performed a study using arthroscopically obtained cartilage biopsies in patients with OA. These biopsy studies may provide a clue as to what newer therapies may work best. Also, they may help in determining the presence of specific genetic markers that may also help us find future treatments.

It also appears that inflammation may have a greater role in OA than previously thought. As noted earlier, IL-1, a potent pro-inflammatory cytokine, seems to be involved in OA. Anti-cytokine drugs may have a role in OA in that these drugs may help modify and alter the course of disease. In fact, they are already being studied as disease-modifying OA drugs.

Other drugs aimed at blocking the effects of destructive enzymes such as matrix metalloproteases also are being explored. Pralnacasan is an inhibitor of interleukin 1 converting enzyme (ICE) and has shown promise in patients with OA.

A broad range of new medications and techniques are currently under study for patients with OA. Among them are the following:

- Nitric oxide, a potent oxidative enzyme that chews up cartilage rapidly, is felt to be a "major player" in OA. Inhibitors of nitric oxide are currently being tested.

- Bone morphogenic protein, a biologic ingredient that appears to promote cartilage growth is undergoing clinical trials.

- Various types of growth factors are being studied on the rationale that certain growth factors may help cartilage regenerate.

- Efforts are under way to find drugs that will modify the structure of cartilage to make it harder and more resilient.

- Genetic factors are being studied that may make it easier to identity patients at risk earlier.

- The participation of the bone underlying cartilage is being explored as well. Perhaps modification of the bone may help cartilage to stay resilient.

- The role of the synovial tissue in starting and perpetuating the inflammation in OA is also being explored. Perhaps the synovium holds the key.

- Minimally invasive surgical procedures in which polymer spacers are inserted to form a cushion inside the joint are being evaluated.

- Minimally invasive surgical techniques where a paste of stem cells and growth factors is inserted into a cartilage defect.

As mentioned earlier, tissue engineering is in its infancy. Perhaps, it may soon be feasible to use a combination of biologically active cells, signal molecules, and a matrix of tissue to hold everything in place. Among these tissue growth stimulation factors are:

- Insulin-like growth factor to stimulate growth of the cartilage matrix
- Fibroblast growth factor to stimulate chondrocyte growth
- Transforming growth factor B to stimulate chondrocytes to grow
- Hepatocyte growth factor to stimulates chondrocytes to make more matrix
- Platelet-derived growth factor to increase matrix synthesis
- Indian hedgehog and parathyroid hormone-related peptide to regulate chondrocyte maturation
- Interleukin-1 receptor antagonist to prevent degradation of cartilage

Stem cell research may hold the key. Because they are capable of regenerating and repairing cartilage, stem cells may serve as "factories" for new cartilage.

At our center, we are actively involved in procedures applying the use of autologous (a patient's own stem cells) stem cells to treat osteoarthritis of the hip and knee. The stem cells are obtained by withdrawing bone marrow from the iliac crest of the pelvis and then concentrating the marrow. We are able to create a concentrate containing approximately five to six million adult stem cells. Using a combination of these stem cells along with growth factors supplied by a patient's own blood and fat to stimulate growth and multiplication of stem cells is a procedure that has worked in animal models.

Our experience to date with this technique in a number of patients with OA involving the knee, shoulder, and hip is very encouraging and there is preliminary evidence that we are able to regenerate some cartilage. For more information about our stem cell procedure, call (301) 694-5800 or go to www.arthritistreatmentcenter.com.

Gene therapy is also being evaluated as a possible system for delivering therapeutic genes. This approach is attractive because it allows the diseased joint to become the site of synthesis of factors for its own repair.

Chapter 6

Conclusion

Osteoarthritis is the most common type of arthritis. It is the result of a premature or excessive wearing away of cartilage. Although multiple palliative treatments are available, there is still no truly effective therapy that addresses the issue of rapid, sustained cartilage regeneration.

This most common form of arthritis is finally getting the attention it deserves. It is my hope that within the next 10 years, we will have specific medicines designed to slow down and even reverse the wear and tear of OA. Within the next few years, we will see a surge in efforts designed to grow and/or make cartilage.

We may even be able to categorize OA using new genotyping techniques. That will allow us to custom-fit therapy!

For more information about arthritis, contact:

The Arthritis Treatment Center

71 Thomas Johnson Drive

Frederick, MD 21702

(301) 694-5800

www.arthritistreatmentcenter.com

www.ingramcontent.com/pod-product-compliance
Lightning Source LLC
Chambersburg PA
CBHW071244170526
45165CB00003B/1232